5:2 Diet

An Amazing Diet for Rapid Weight Loss to Enhance Your Health (Salad Recipes, Vegan Recipes, Low Carb Recipes; Weight Loss Books)

By Jennifer DeMoines

Table of Contents

Introduction

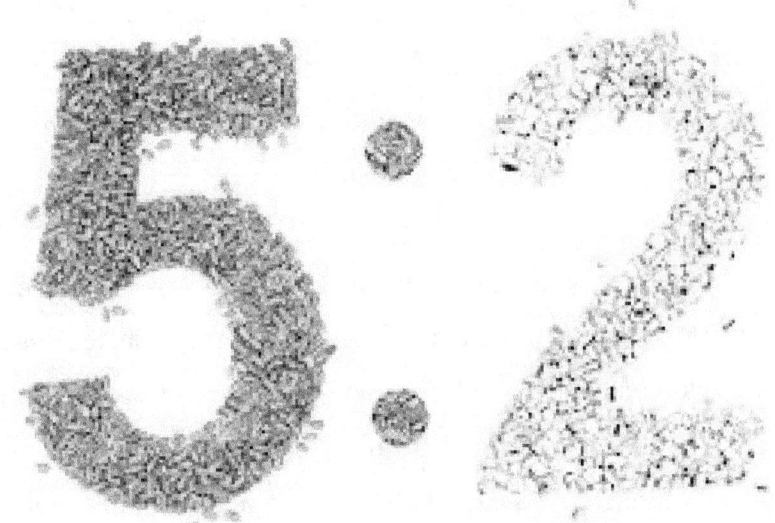

We all know the Hippocrates belief "Your food is your first medicine", and it's definitely a true statement that is repeated for more than two thousand years. The modern way of life brought us lots of benefits but in the same time, our nutritional habits became worse than ever. Processed food, numerous added ingredients in almost all food products, unfortunately, took its price – our health. So, what can we do to retain our well-being? The Internet is flooded with a number of diets, books, articles about special kinds of diets and all of them promise wonders in a just a few days. So, why is this particular diet I want to present you different from others? First of all, this diet was created by two scientists, Dr. Michelle Harvie, nutrition specialist, and Dr. Tony Howell, oncologist, and it is intended for all those who love and enjoy every bite and still look good – without a pound of extra weight. Diet 5:2 did not result from unverified theory, but it is a result of scientific research that started in 2006 at the Institute Genesis Breast Cancer Prevention in Manchester, UK.

In this book, you will find everything that you need to know about 5:2 diet. Firstly, you need to know that with fasting of just 2 days weekly you will not just achieve your weight goal but you will also boost your immune system, keeping insulin levels in balance in your bloodstream, speed up metabolism and above all this, this diet will preserve all your muscle and help you lose the fat around your belly. Fasting as a temporary or permanent waiver of certain food habit is present in various forms, in all religions, and throughout the history of mankind from prehistory time. Many kinds of fasting are present nowadays and had been held in the various religions before Christianity. Greek writer Herodotus (known as the father of history) stated that even ancient Egyptians fasted once a month to preserve health and youth. A book called "Basic principles of medical science" that dates back to the fourth century BC, Tibet, contains a special chapter dedicated to link and treatment between food and fasting.

Besides Christians, fasting was practiced among Jews, Muslims, Confucianism, Hindus, Taoists, Jains and many other religious groups. The length of fasting differs in each religion from 1 up to 40 days. Today fasting doesn't have to be only on the religious base, but every individual can decide to do it on their own or in a number of clinics around the world. The positive effects of fasting are:

> natural detoxification,
> decomposition of energy reserves (which is stored in fatty tissue)
> successful treatment of many metabolic diseases or disorders whose source is poor diet,
> It helps in preservation of physical and mental abilities,
> It helps with weight loss and rejuvenation (skin becomes smooth and shiny)

We could freely say that periodical fasting brings many benefits to our body overall.

Chapter 1: Why is fasting so crucial in diet 5:2

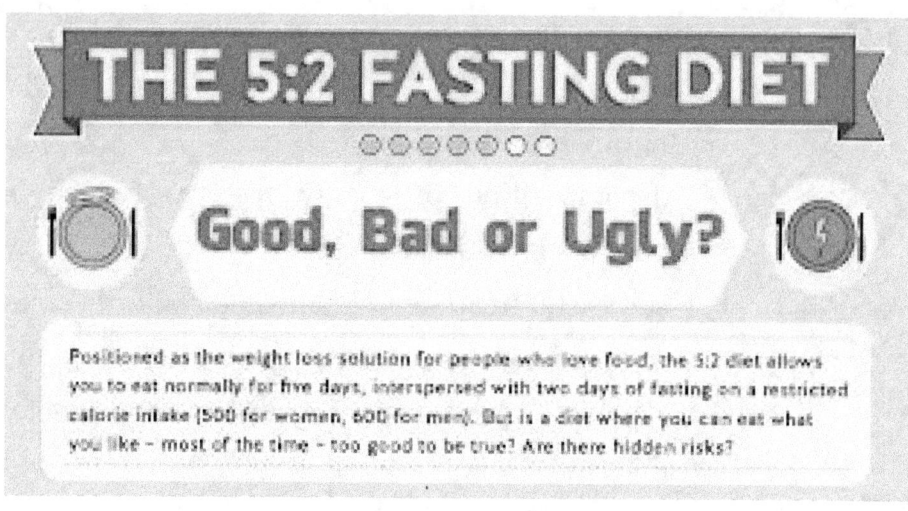

THE 5:2 FASTING DIET

Good, Bad or Ugly?

Positioned as the weight loss solution for people who love food, the 5:2 diet allows you to eat normally for five days, interspersed with two days of fasting on a restricted calorie intake (500 for women, 600 for men). But is a diet where you can eat what you like - most of the time - too good to be true? Are there hidden risks?

This diet is based on simple rules and it's not overly restrictive, which means that it allows longer following than any other limiting kinds of diets. Why? Simply, because you need to restrict your daily intake of food for just two days during a week, but nevertheless it doesn't mean that you can overeat for the rest of the week. During fasting period most people conduct vegetarian or Mediterranean kind of cuisine.

Fasting is needed mostly because of the presence and accumulation of toxins (poisons) in the blood, cells, brain, bones, glands, skin, or rather in all our tissues, causing a weakening of the immune system and lowers the ability of proper operation of all organs in our body. We intake some toxins in our body through food and some of them are produced by our own body during metabolism processes. As everything else in our life, balance is crucial and for our body, it means that we need to keep our acid-alkaline balance ratio equal. The condition of pH of the human body may be measured through saliva, blood or urine. If our body is more acidly, it leads to premature aging , it can cause many health problems, diseases as cancers and even lead to death.

Fasting is the quickest way of detoxification process and elimination of toxins from our body. Maintaining a healthy body weight is one of the most important factors if you want to avoid any of many health problems (physical and mental), and each of us can affect on it.

You need to know that if your goal is weight loss then you need to restrict your calorie intake for at least 25% so your body could start to use wasting mass as an energy source. But, carried out by research Dr. Michelle Harvie and Dr. Tony Howell showed that the 2-Day Diet during a week is more effective, harmless, practical, and overall it showed a higher rate of weight loss compared to daily dieting.

Keeping a strict diet twice a week can be the key to successful weight loss.

How does it work? Whenever we consume food, our body needs to act fast so it could be able to regulate the sudden overflow of glucose we entered into our systems during digestion. With the first bite, you take, a hormone known as insulin is released so it could "take up" glucose from our blood and store it in our liver, muscles and fat tissue. When you restrict your food intake, insulin won't be released in your bloodstream and levels of glucose in the blood will stay stable. Our body can't use fat as an energy source while insulin levels are high, and that happens every time you eat because glucose levels rise. Many short-term starvation studies have proven that levels of glucose in the blood fall during starvation. Only then our body responds and uses fat as the main energy source so our body could carry out all functions (breathing, muscle moving including normal heart function.) This all happens within 14 hours after the last meal.

This diet works on the following principle: choose any two days per week and restrict food intake during those days. Women are allowed to intake between 500 kcal and men 600 kcal per day but not more than 1000 calories. My advice is that you should do it on Monday and Thursday, because weekend just ended and on Monday you are probably still full of energy because you had time to "fill your batteries" during the weekend, and Thursday is better to choose than Friday because most of us hardly wait for Friday to relax or spend time with your family or friends. It is important that the days you choose do not follow one another, but that there is a gap of at least 24 hours between them. Nevertheless, each of us has our own schedule and after all, it doesn't matter which two days you choose for fasting, what is important is that you stick to them.

What to eat during fasting days

I will tell you first what you **can't eat** during your fasting days. Among forbidden food are bread, cereals, starch, legumes, take away food, processed meals, bad fats, and simple sugar. Now, you are probably scratching your head and asking yourself "what the heck will I eat during those days, I will starve". Don't worry, there are a plenty of food that you can eat. You can eat raw or steamed vegetables, dairy products from partially skimmed milk and proteins from eggs, nuts, fish and lean meat.

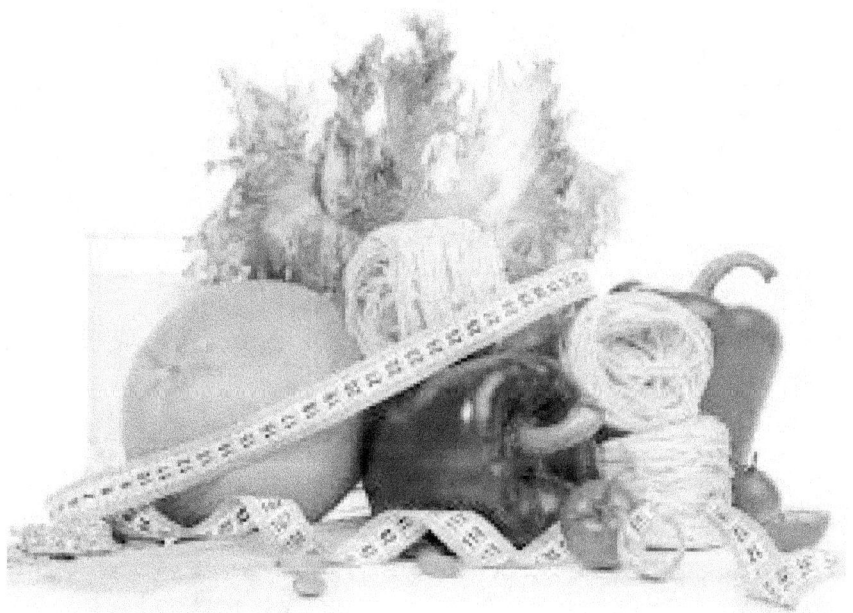

Proven benefits of food taken during fasting

Our body is full of "good" and" bad" bacteria, that exist in our digestive tract. Their aim assignment is to break down food and turn it into energy needed for normal functioning of our organism.

Food like ***dairy products*** contain natural probiotics (good bacteria that live in our guts) so during fasting days it's important to intake more dairy products and so "raise" the level of good bacteria with the purpose of helping with better digestion and achieving much faster slimming. Below are ingredients that you should choose during your fasting days, as a part of breakfast or dinner meals.

Food	amount	kcal	proteins	fats	carbs	dietary fibers
Greek yogurt	1 container (170g)	100	17.32	0.66	6.12	0
Feta cheese	1 oz (28.35g)	75	4.03	6.03	1.16	0
cream cheese	1 tbsp.	35	0.62	3.44	0.55	0
mozzarella nonfat	half a cup (56g)	80	17.91	0	1.98	1

food	Amount	kcal	proteins	fats	carbs	dietary fibers
kefir low fat	1 cup (250g)	102	9.48	2.32	11.2	0

Seed like pumpkin, sesame, sunflower, flax, caraway (cumin) are full of antioxidants, soluble fibers, and omega-3 fatty acids. They also contain essential minerals such as calcium, magnesium, copper, and iron. The best way to use them is to roast them gently under light heat. You need to ground some of them like flaxseeds and caraway, before using them in a recipe, (otherwise your body won't be able to use soluble fibers from them).

food	Amount	kcal	proteins	fats	carbs	dietary fibers
sesame seeds, dried	1 tbsp.	52	1.6	4.47	2.11	1.1
Pumpkin seeds	1 tbsp.	65	3.38	5.56	1.67	0.7
flaxseeds	1 tbsp. ground	37	1.28	2.95	2.02	1.09
sunflower seeds with hulls	handful	27	0.96	2.37	0.92	0.4
sunflower seeds no hulls	handful	49	1.64	4.24	2.05	0.9
caraway seeds (spice)	1 tbsp.	22	1.32	0.98	3.34	2.5

**Eggs** – are also an excellent choice of food during fasting days because they contain almost all essential amino acids. Without them, our body wouldn't be able to perform any life process, and they are absolutely essential for every metabolic process. We can freely say that eggs belong to the so- called "super food" or as I rather say functional food because they contain a little bit of almost every nutrient our body needs. You shouldn't be worried too much about cholesterol content in them because one medium egg contains about 100mg of cholesterol that presents just a third of recommended daily limit which is 300mg. Cholesterol (a type of fat), is one natural component of blood and our body produces almost 75% of all daily needs of it.

Many researchers suggest that if you habitually eat eggs for breakfast you will even reduce the risk of heart attack.

food	amount	kcal	proteins	fats	carbs	dietary fibers
egg cooked	large	90	6.26	6.83	0.38	0
egg omelet	large	94	6.45	7.11	0.39	0
egg poached	medium	72	6.26	4.74	0.36	0
egg powder	1 tbsp.	44	5.49	1.29	2.16	0

**Fish** - especially fatty fish contains high amounts of essential unsaturated omega 3 fatty acids that our body cannot create. Our body needs them to stay healthy because they have a crucial role in proper function of our nervous, cardiovascular and immune systems. Without omega 3 fatty acids our body simply cannot work.

food	amount	kcal	proteins	fats	carbs	dietary fibers
Cod, Hake cooked	half fillet 3 oz (90g)	94	20.55	0.77	0	0
Trout cooked	1 fillet 2.5 oz (70g)	119	16,9	5,14	0	0
tuna canned in water	1 can (165g)	142	32.8	1,58	0	0
Sardine in tomato sauce	1 piece	70	7,93	3,97	0,21	0
sardine canned in oil	2 pieces	50	5,91	2,75	0	0
Tilapia, cooked,	1 fillet 3 oz (85g)	111	22,75	2,31	0	0

Poultry meat is also one excellent choice when you are on your fasting days because those are the days when your body is under the impact of stress and poultry contains two very valuable nutrients that are great for reducing stress – tryptophan (essential kind of amino acid) and Vitamin B5. Those nutrients have a calming effect on your nervous system and this makes poultry an excellent option when you are fasting. They also contain a high amount of proteins, and more proteins provide longer satiety filling during a day.

food	amount	kcal	proteins	fats	carbs	dietary fibers
Turkey white meat roasted	1 serving 3 oz (85g)	125	25,61	1,77	0	0
Chicken white meat roasted	3 oz (85g)	94	17,28	2,3	0	0

Dark green veggies and cabbage sort should be on your menu during fasting days because they contain a higher amount of dietary fibers that also gives us satiety feeling and you won't be hungry during a day which is the point. But it would be good if those ingredients are more present in your meals during the whole week and not just fasting days. You can see the pattern that can be implied for all veggies below: Low caloric content, high fiber content.

food	amount	kcal	proteins	fats	carbs	dietary fibers
Broccoli, raw	1 cup	31	2,57	0,34	6,04	2,4
Brussels sprouts, cooked,	10 sprouts	76	5,36	1,05	14,91	5,5
Spinach	1 cup chopped	45	5,66	0,89	6,57	4,5
Beans, snap, green,	10 beans 4" long	17	1	0,12	3,83	1,5
Peas green	1 cup	117	7,86	0,58	20,95	8,3
Lettuce salad	1 cup	8	0,58	0,1	1,55	1
Collards leaf	1 cup chopped	12	1,09	0,22	1,95	1,4
Cabbage, raw	1 cup chopped	22	1,14	0,09	5,16	2,2

__Fruits__ – I suppose that everyone knows that fruits are loaded with antioxidants (compounds that act protectively in our organism) and that they are naturally short in calories although they are very rich in fibers, and all others vital nutrients like vitamins, omega 3 fatty acids (nuts). Nevertheless, I need to remind you that fruit in dried form such as apricots, prunes, raisins, figs etc. are more concentrated in calories than in fresh form so, you need to consume them in smaller amounts.

food	Amount	kcal	proteins	fats	carbs	dietary fibers
Apple, 3" dia.	medium size 160g	77	0.43	0.21	20.54	2.1
Pears	small size 150g	84	0.53	0.21	22.54	4.6
Orange	medium size 150g	69	1.06	0.32	17.43	3.6
Bananas	medium size 120g	105	1.29	0.39	26.95	3.1
Prune	1 pitted	23	0.21	0.04	6.07	0.7
Raisins, seedless	a handful	62	0.64	0.1	16.47	0.8
Apricot dried	3 halves	25	0.36	0.05	6.58	0.8
Almonds roasted	11 pieces	86	3.01	7.82	2.51	1.5
Walnuts	7 halves	93	2.16	9.24	1.94	0.9

When you are on your fasting days, don't forget that you should intake more liquid so that detoxification process is performed more efficiency. I don't mean that you need to drink a gallon of water but it would be good that you stick to recommended amounts of 8 cups for women and 10 cups for men on those days. Don't worry, you won't be overloaded with liquids if you enter even 12 cups of preferably tap water during a day because on average base we lose about 2l of water (this refers to people who don't do much exercise and during not so sunny days), athletes lose much more. When we talk about beverages it would be better that you restrict soda drinks intake, especially during fasting days, because they are loaded with hidden sugars.

Chapter 2: Some recipes during fasting days

Even so that many believe that buckwheat belongs to cereals; it is actually a fruit seed so you can use it in your breakfast meals during fasting days. Two tablespoons of raw buckwheat Groats contains only 19 calories.

Spiced Buckwheat &apple

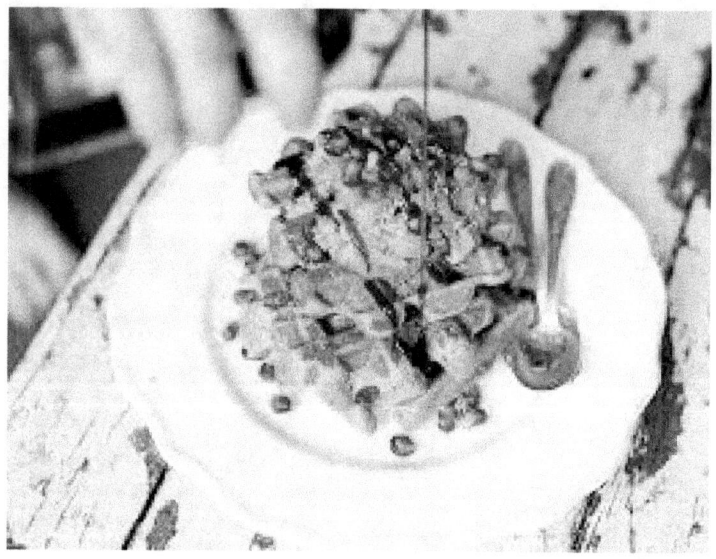

Breakfast

No. of Serves: 1

Preparation time 5 minutes, provided with the buckwheat that submerged in water over the night.

Cooking time: 15 minutes

Ingredients:

- 2 tbsp. of roasted buckwheat Groats,
- 1 shredded medium sized apple
- 1 tsp. of cinnamon

Preparation:

1. Cook buckwheat in a boiling water (a cup of water will be enough)
2. Drain it. Add shredded apple and cinnamon. Serve

Nutritional Facts: this meal contains **120 calories**; 0.5g of fat; 31.2 g of carbs; 6.2 g of dietary fibers and 1.3g of proteins. Good points are that this meal is very low in saturated fats, no cholesterol, very low in sodium, very high in dietary fibers, high in manganese and very high in vitamin B6 and C.

Salmon and broccoli flowerets baked in foil

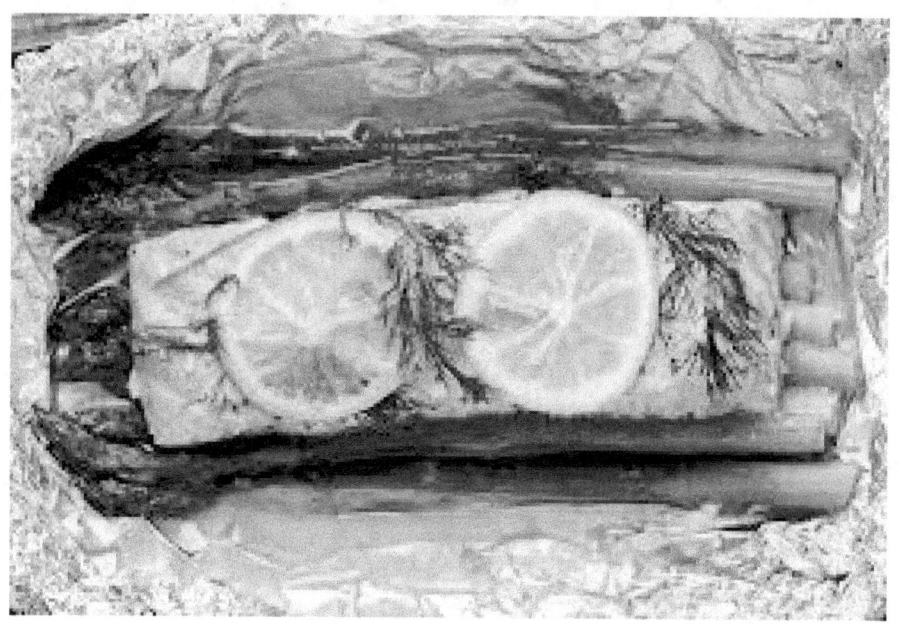

Lunch

No. of Serves: 1

Preparation time: 20 minutes:

Cooking time: 25 minutes

Ingredients:

- 2 tbsp. of fresh parsley
- 3 mint leaves
- ¼ of a tsp. of sea salt
- 1 crushed garlic clove

- ¼ of a tsp. of sweet dried red pepper spice
- 2 tbsp of fresh lemon juice
- 1 tbsp of olive oil.
- 3 oz of salmon fillet
- A cup of chopped broccoli flowerets

Preparation:

1. Preheat the oven to 430°F or 220°C.

2. Blend parsley and mint leaves, salt, garlic together in a food processor to make a rough paste. Add the lemon juice, dried red pepper and process until fairly smooth. Spoon over the sauce into a bowl and combine with the salmon, then marinate for 20 minutes.

3. Place the marinated fish in the center of the foil, line over the broccoli, wrap the ends of the foil to form a spiral shape so that it's completely sealed and no steam can escape.

4. Place the foil packet on the baking sheet. Bake for about 25 minutes. Serve

Nutritional Facts: this meal contains **293 calories**; 19.6g of fat; 6.5 g of carbs; 3.0 g of dietary fibers and 18.4 g of proteins. Good points are that this meal is very low in sodium, high in magnesium, phosphorus, and selenium. Selenium has antioxidant properties like vitamin C does, so it would be good that this meal is on your table at least once a week.

Tomato soup with carrot and flaxseeds

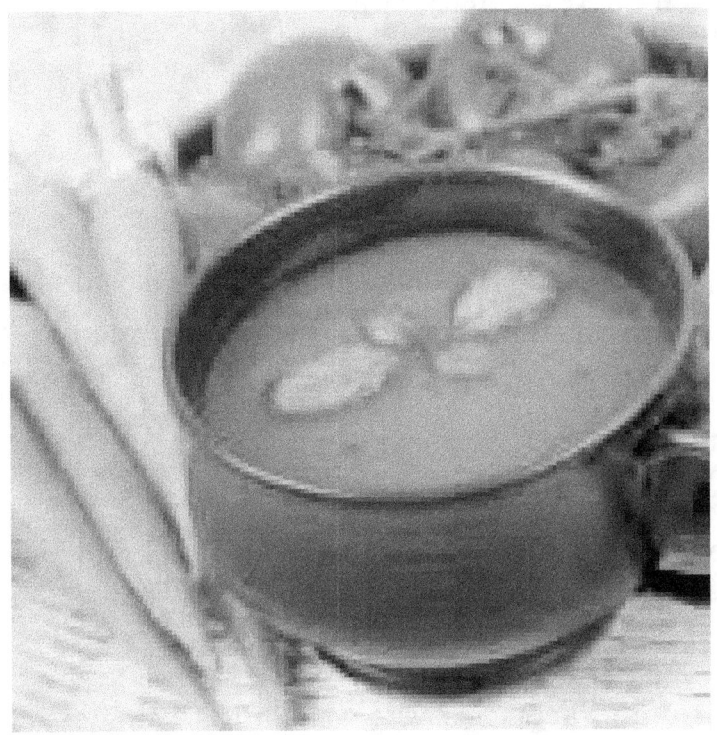

No. of Serves: 1

Preparation time: 10 minutes:

Cooking time: 10 minutes

<u>Ingredients for 4 servings</u>:

- 1 medium chopped carrot
- 2 tbsp of a parsley root
- ½ a cup of crushed canned tomatoes,

- 1 tbsp. of Flaxseed
- 2 cups of water
- 1 tbsp. fresh parsley,
- pinch of salt
- pinch of pepper

Preparation:

1. Put all chopped veggies (carrot, parsley root, and tomatoes) in a saucepan on the stove over medium heat. Add just a bit of water. Cook for about 2 minutes, then stir with tbsp. of grounded flax seeds, mix everything together nicely and pour the rest of water immediately.

2. Let it cook for about 10 minutes until veggies are tender.

3. Turn off the stove and add spices. Serve.

Nutritional Facts: this soup contains **85 calories**; 2.8 g of fat; 12.8 g of carbs; 4.8 g of dietary fibers and 3.3 g of proteins. Good points are that this soup is low in saturated fat, it doesn't contain cholesterol and what is important it has a high content of dietary fibers so it will clean your guts and it contains antioxidants in the form of vitamins A and C.

This whole meal plan day contains **498 calories, 22.9** g of fat; **50.5** g of carbs of whom **14** g are dietary fibers and **23** g of proteins. This means that your liver, kidneys and guts have time to "recover" because they won't have to deal with a large number of artificial ingredients that we usually intake with our common diet.

Fake Granola bars

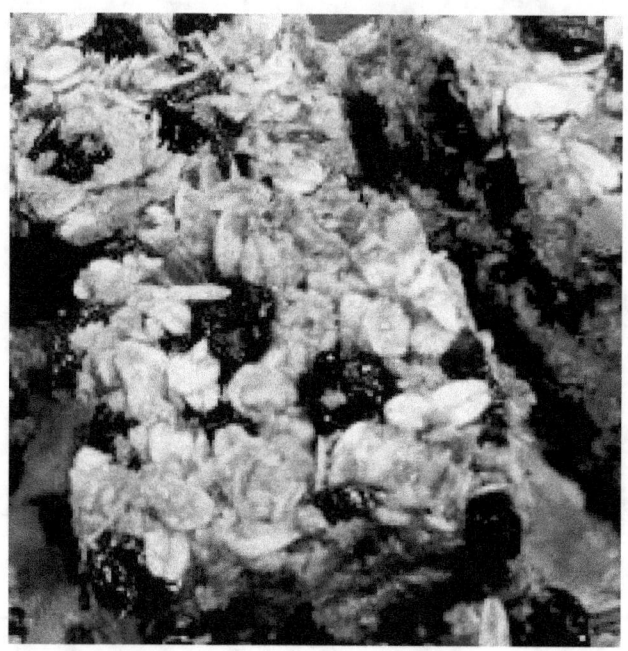

Breakfast

No. of Serves: 8

Preparation time 10 minutes.

Cooking time: 10 -15 minutes

Ingredients:

- 1 cup of roasted buckwheat grounded a bit
- 2 cups of grated and chopped apple,
- 1 freshly squeezed orange
- 1 tsp. of flax seed

- 1 tsp. of sunflower seeds
- 1 tbsp. of cinnamon
- Almond flour to make this all thicken (1-2 tablespoon).

Preparation:

1. Mix all dry ingredients thoroughly, add orange juice and line the "batter" in an 8X8 inch baking pan with parchment paper
2. With an extra sheet of parchment paper, press down the mixture to close it and assure there are no spaces in the "batter" and bake in the oven at 350°F -180°C for 10 to 15 minutes.
3. Remove parchment paper from the pan and cut with a knife, slice into 8 even bars.

Nutritional Facts: one bar contains only **122 calories**; 2.7g of fat; 23.4 g of carbs; 4.3 g of dietary fibers and 3.6 g of proteins. Good points are that each bar is very low in saturated fats, no cholesterol, very low in sodium, very high in dietary fibers, high in manganese and magnesium and very high in vitamin B6 and C.

Walnut Cabbage salad

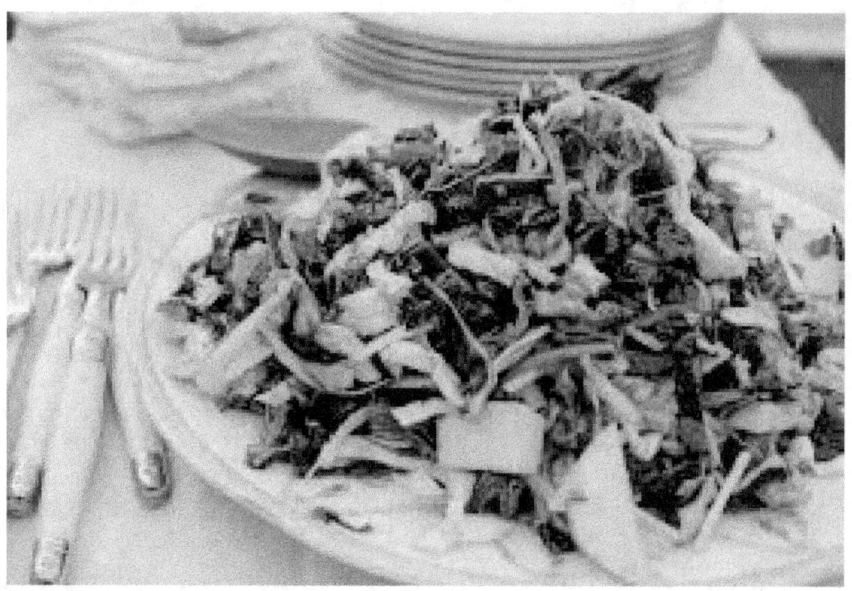

Lunch

No. of Serves: 1

Preparation time: 10 minutes:

Cooking time: none

Ingredients:

- 1 cup of shredded white cabbage
- 1 cup of shredded red cabbage
- 1 medium sliced carrot
- 1 chopped medium sized green apple
- 4 halves of coarsely chopped walnuts

Dressing:

- Juice of half a lemon
- 1 tsp. of Extra Virgin Olive Oil
- Pinch of sea salt.

Preparation: mix all ingredients. Spice the salad.

Nutritional Facts: this salad contains **161 calories**; 6.2 g of fat; 28.3 g of carbs; 6.7 g of dietary fibers and 2.1 g of proteins. Good points are that this salad is high in dietary fibers and it contains powerful antioxidants in the form of vitamins and essential omega 3 fatty acids. Especially nuts content influence on reducing the risk of getting diabetes, but be beware that they are very caloric so you should consume them in moderation amount (few pieces each day).

Stewed Spinach with sesame seeds

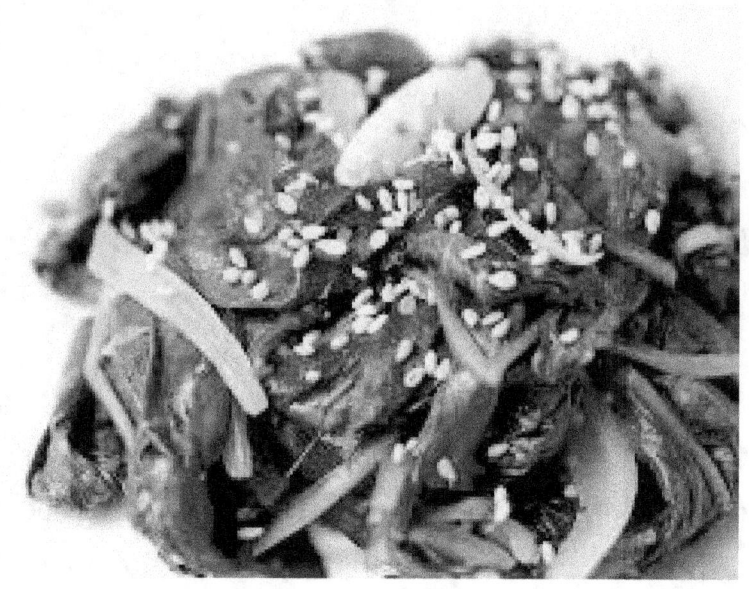

No. of Serves: 1

Preparation time: 5 minutes

Cooking time: 10 minutes

Ingredients:

- 2 cups of spinach,
- 2 tbsp. of roasted and grounded sesame seeds,
- ¼ of a cup of milk
- 1 tsp. of butter
- Pinch of salt
- 1 tbsp of Greek yogurt

Preparation:

1. Grind the sesame seeds in a blender.
2. Put spinach in boiling water for a few seconds, put it aside to cool and drain. Add milk, a little salt, and crushed sesame seeds and stir well. It goes great with Greek yogurt or sour cream.

Nutritional Facts: this salad contains **244 calories**; 17.5 g of fat; 10.5 g of carbs; 5.2 g of dietary fibers and 9.4 g of proteins. Good points are that this stew is low in cholesterol and sugar, but it is very high in calcium, iron, manganese, magnesium. I need to mention that our body loses minerals such as calcium and magnesium when we are under the impact of stress. This means that this meal provides for our body with minerals so that the stress impact to which we are exposed will, at least, be alleviated a bit.

This whole meal plan day contains **527 calories, 26.4** g of fat; **62.2** g of carbs of whom **16.2** g are dietary fibers and **15.1** g of proteins. Even thou this day is based on a vegetarian diet you will enter a minimum of requested proteins and so avoid muscle loss during fasting.

Boiled egg with cream cheese and pumpkin seeds spread

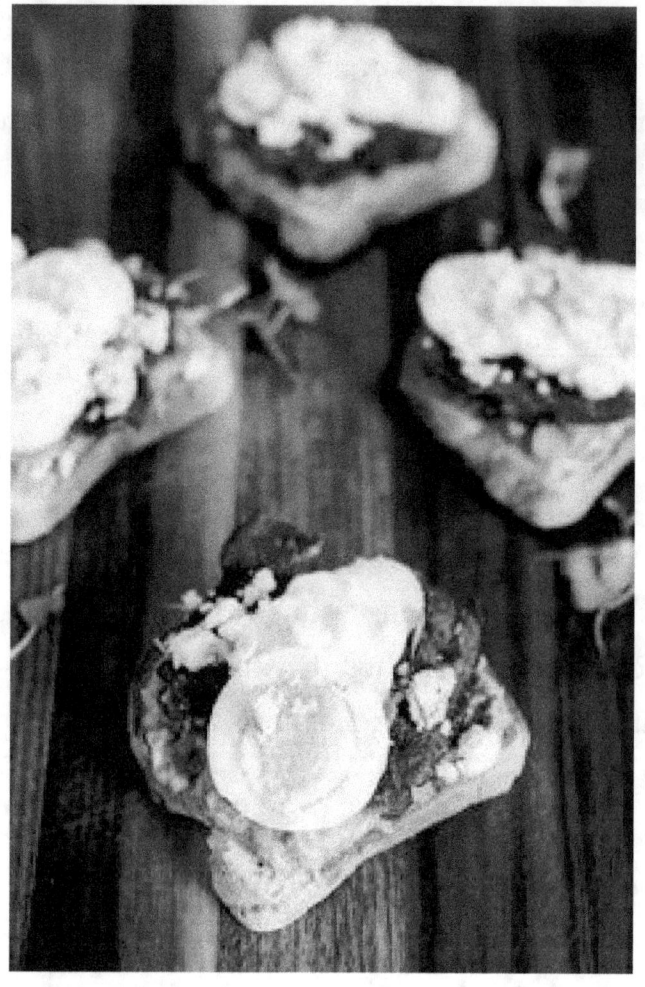

Breakfast

No. of Serves: 1

Preparation time 5 minutes.

Cooking time: 8 minutes

Ingredients:

- 1 hardboiled egg
- 1 tsp. of cream cheese
- 1 tsp. of pumpkin seeds, coarsely chopped
- 1 outer lettuce leaf

Preparation:

1. Cook the egg in boiling water
2. Mix roasted pumpkin seeds with cream cheese.
3. Wash lettuce leaf, spread it and pour over cream cheese with seeds.
4. Cut boiled egg into rings, spread it over and roll lettuce leaf into a roll. Serve.

Nutritional Facts: This breakfast contains only **94 calories**; 7.0 g of fat; 1.5 g of carbs; 0.5 g of dietary fibers and 6.5 g of proteins. Good points are that this meal contains low sugar content (or as I like to call them empty carbs), high in phosphorus high in riboflavin, very high in selenium and very high in vitamins A and B12.

Stuffed tomatoes with egg, cream cheese & raisins

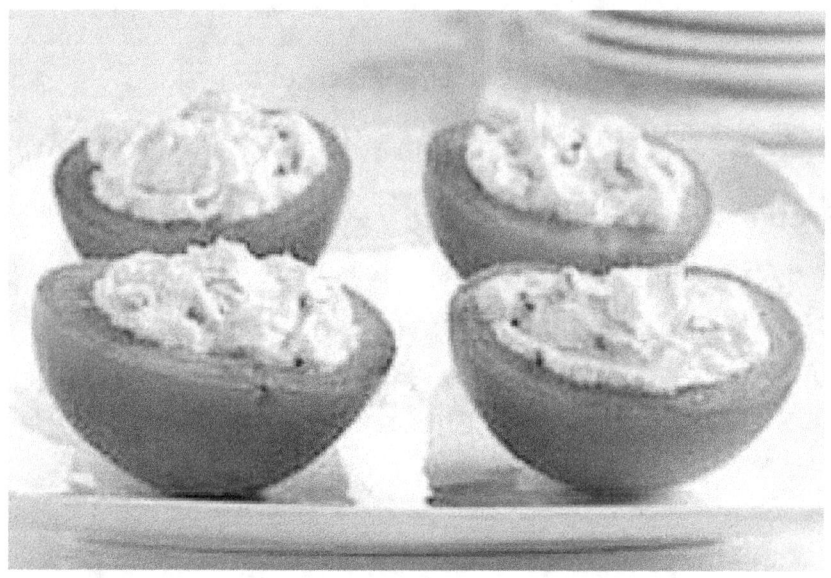

Lunch

No. of Serves: 1

Preparation time 5 minutes.

Cooking time: 15 minutes

Ingredients:

- 1 large tomato
- 1 tbsp. of chopped ginger
- 1 tbsp. of cream cheese
- 1 tbsp. of golden dry raisins
- 1 egg

Preparation:

1. Wash tomato, and cut off upper part.
2. Preheat the oven to 356°F or 180°C or cook it in a microwave for 5 minutes.
3. Put the "lid" of the tomato aside. With a small spoon dug tomato from the inside.
4. Mix ginger with the crushed tomatoes and raisins, which had previously been submerged in water for 10 minutes.
5. Add cream cheese, mix all and fill hollowed tomato with a spoon, add cracked egg and cover with "lid" of the tomato.
6. Put stuffed tomato into the previously greased baking pan. Bake it for about 15 minutes at 200 ° C – 390° F - until it becomes brown or you can cook it much faster in a microwave.

Nutritional Facts: This meal contains only **149 calories**; 8.5 g of fat; 11.5 g of carbs; 2.9 g of dietary fibers and 8.4 g of proteins. Good points are that this meal is high in potassium, high in manganese and selenium, very high in vitamins A and C.

Grilled chicken and Arugula &zucchini puree

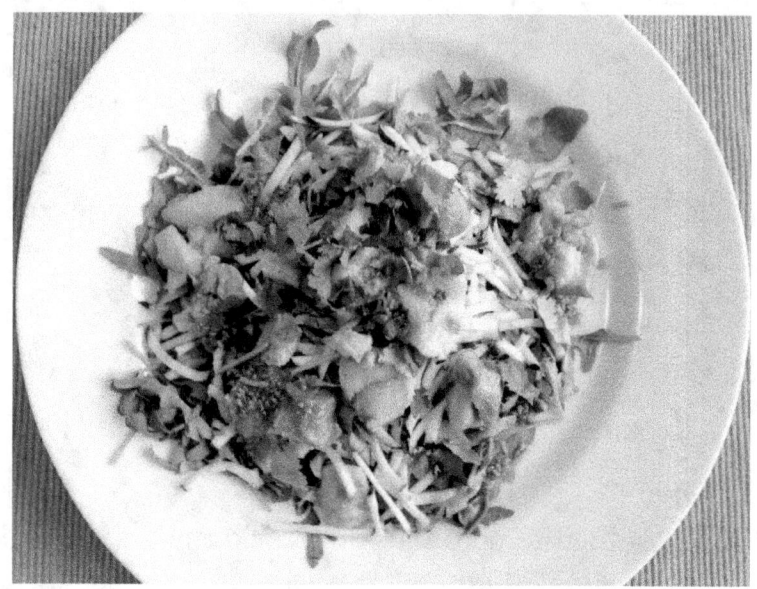

Dinner

No. of Serves: 1

Preparation time 10 minutes; and 1 hour for the chicken to rest in the marinade.

Cooking time: 15 minutes

Ingredients:

- 1 tbsp. of dried oregano
- 1 tsp. of olive oil
- 2 tbsp. of freshly squeezed lemon juice
- 3 oz of chicken breast (make two slices)

- 1 cup of arugula
- 1 small zucchini
- 1 tsp. of dill
- 2 cloves of chopped garlic
- 1 tsp. of olive oil

Preparation:

1. Combine oil, lemon juice and oregano in a mixing bowl. Pour over chicken steak and leave it in a fridge for at least an hour.

2. Preheat the grill to medium heat and lightly spread with oil.

3. Place chicken on the grill and cook until lightly browned and cooked through, it takes about 5 minutes if it's thinner. Turn chicken over and cook until it gets a well-browned color.

4. Pour a cup of water in saucepan to boil and then add washed arugula and peeled and chopped zucchini into small pieces. Cook for a few minutes, drain and make a puree with stick blender. Add a bit of dill, salt, olive oil, and garlic. Serve with grilled chicken.

Nutritional Facts: This meal contains only **276 calories**; 13.5 g of fat; 10.8 g of carbs; 3.9 g of dietary fibers and 30.6 g of proteins. Good points are that this meal contains very high content of niacin, vitamin B12. Niacin belongs to vitamin B groups and its one powerful ant-inflammatory nutrient.

This whole meal plan day contains **519 calories, 29** g of fat; **23.8** g of carbs of whom **7.3** g are dietary fibers and **45.5** g of proteins.

During other 5 days, it would be good that you avoid processed ready to serve meals as much as possible. If you are dining out order portion for kids and try to eat as slowly as you can. This is very important because our brain sends a signal of satiety after 20 minutes from the moment when we start eating.

Another trick to speed up your metabolism is to drink water before each main meal, especially colder water. In one of many researches that were done, 84 obesity people participated during 12 weeks. They had to drink 2 cups (500 ml) of water half an hour before their main meals. Participants who drank that amount of water lost two pounds (1.2 kg), more than participants who didn't drink water half an hour before each meal.

Whenever you can, buy organic groceries especially when you are buying fresh veggies and fruits. This is important because ingredients that are treated with pesticides will make your main goal when it comes to weight loss much harder to reach, but this isn't the worst news. The longer impact of pesticides leads to many neurodegenerative disorders such as Parkinson diseases, Alzheimer and overall lack of many mental abilities (including lack of concentration, sleeping disorders and so on). You need to be aware that it is necessary to wash fruits and vegetables primarily in any case because of bacteria, germs, and other natural contaminants. It is also possible to wash some kinds of pesticides with water, but you can't wash all of them.

Another advice is that during non-fasting days you eat more proteins (lean meat, eggs, dairy products and legumes).

You can prepare nice yummy shakes and smoothies as snacks, eat a handful of berries, or dried fruits and nuts (only 2 -3 pieces). Make some muffins with a healthier choice of ingredients. Instead of simple sugar or artificial sweetener, you should use organic honey.

Conclusion

For conclusion, I would remind you that fasting is needed mostly because of the presence and accumulation of toxins (poisons) in our body. Fasting was practiced from the prehistoric period so it's definitely proven as one of the best methods if you want to stay healthy and good looking. I really think those 2 days of fasting during a week aren't a too big sacrifice if you know that you will not only lose some extra pounds but in the same time, you will increase your mental and physical abilities.

That's why I have provided you with a small nutritional table contest with the most common ingredients that are usually used during fasting days. This way, you will easily calculate the calorie intake and then prepare meals which suit you best.

As my last advice for rest of the week, when it comes to dieting I would recommend you to uphold Mediterranean cuisine because this is one of the best and healthiest ways for preparing food. This kind of diet offers you a lot of healthy ingredients and what is more important when we are talking about properly preparing food, Mediterranean nutrition provides you meals with the most valuable nutrients preserved.

Don't forget to exercise at least twice a week and find a way to relax from everyday stress.

www.ingramcontent.com/pod-product-compliance
Lightning Source LLC
Chambersburg PA
CBHW071144280526
45787CB00003B/1395